50 Foods to avoid to Lose weight and Stay Happy and Healthy

I0416874

By Malik Johnson

Table of Contents

Introduction

NOT just another diet book

If you're reading this right now, you, like millions of people around the world, have probably tried to shed unwanted weight and feel healthier and happier. Maybe you've tried several diets and you're skeptical, because no matter what kind of diet you followed or how hard you tried, none of them ever really worked like they promised. Well, I've got a secret that I need to share with you: NONE OF THEM EVER WILL!

That's because conventional diets-the ones we've all heard about, the ones that are supposed to be the solution to all our weight problems- are the

REAL problem. Conventional diets are all too often jam-packed with supposedly "healthy" foods that are actually causing all the weight gain, health problems and even mood disorders in the first place! As long as you keep eating these secretly toxic foods, you'll be on the hamster wheel of health, spinning and spinning, trying to change your weight and health for the better and NEVER GETTING ANYWHERE.

This book and the information it will give you is NOT just another ordinary diet book. It is a powerful tool that will help you break the cycle of diet after unsuccessful diet, get you off that hamster wheel for good and put you back in control of your weight, your health and your happiness. This book will change the way you think about food, the way you eat and ultimately, it will change the way you look, feel and live. Are you ready to find out which dead foods have been secretly sabotaging your health? Do you want to learn the shocking secret that's making you sick, fat and depressed? How about finding out about the amazing enzymes that can help you start shedding pounds and feeling fit, strong and fantastic from this moment on? If the answer is yes, yes and yes, you're about to unlock the door to fitness, health and happiness.

How This Book Works:

This book has several very important messages, including:

- Message # 1: "Know Your Enemy."

- Message # 2: "Eliminate and Replace."

- Message #3: "Bad for the Belly, Bad for the Brain"
- And Much, Much More!

The first message will help you to identify the 50 foods you absolutely must avoid to lose weight and stay healthy and happy. These 50 foods are probably in your fridge and cupboards right now. Maybe you're munching on some of them as you read this. Perhaps you've even been told how healthy and good for you they are. No matter what the packaging says, these nutritionally dead foods can never give you the life affirming vigor and health you need. With this book, you'll be able to target and eliminate the health vampires that are literally sucking the vitality and fitness out of your body with every bite you take.

Once you know what to eliminate from your diet, you'll need to choose a replacement. It's easy to toss out bad foods but if you don't know what to eat instead, you'll definitely lose the battle. That's where message # 2 comes in. This book will show you how to kick the toxic, weight gain causing, health sapping foods to the curb AND how to replace them with living, revitalizing, nourishing foods that will start changing your body and life almost immediately.

But it's not just about your body. This book also focuses on the mind-body connection with message #3. Whatever toxins you ingest, they will have an equally negative impact on the belly AND the brain. Research has shown that weight loss is excellent for brain health and mood stability. This book will point out how to eat to avoid happiness-destroying junk and replace it with whole, real foods that will lighten your body and light up your brain.

With important nutritional information, weight-loss increasing and health and mood boosting tips and delicious, vitality-boosting smoothie recipes included, this book will take you from the very first step all the way to the moment that you realize you have achieved your goals and won the battle to lose weight and stay healthy and happy!

It may seem difficult at times to toss out everything you thought you knew about health and weight loss but here's my advice: If you keep doing what you've always done, you'll keep getting what you've always gotten.

If you still haven't had the great results you want with all the past diets and methods you've tried, why keep doing what you've always done? The information in this book is different. It will challenge you and push you but at the end it will give you a whole new start.

Are you ready to change your life? Then join me in Chapter 1 to find out about some of the so-called "healthy" foods that have been secretly sabotaging your weight and well-being. Let's go!

Chapter 1

Ditch the Dead Stuff!

How to stop killing your food and start saving your life

Imagine for a moment that I gave you a powerful "Secret Nutritional Ingredient" that could heal, repair and boost your body, help you quickly loose unwanted weight and even improve your mind and your mood. What would you do with it? Would you try to swallow it immediately? Or would you throw it into a burning fire and then try to eat it?

I know what you're thinking. What a silly question! Of course you'd never burn something so precious and valuable. Right?

Wrong! If you've ever eaten well-cooked vegetables, legumes and fruits, you've already thrown that "precious ingredient" into a burning fire. How? Well, foods in their natural state contain powerful substances called enzymes. These enzymes are almost miraculously good for us. They do everything from preventing fat and toxins from being stored in our bodies to giving us great digestion, healthy glowing skin, fighting deadly diseases like cancer and heart disease, improving our moods and minds to helping us add years to our lives. They almost sound too good to be true! So what's the catch?

Every time we cook foods over 116 degrees Fahrenheit, we totally burn these life-giving enzymes. Once food is cooked beyond this point, the enzymes are completely destroyed and the food we're left with is no longer living, healthy food that increases our vitality. Instead it becomes cooked, zapped, dead food that in turn zaps our bodies and minds, literally destroying us the way we destroyed those enzymes! In fact, according to enzyme expert Dr. Edward Howell (author of *Food Enzymes for Health and Longevity*), eating mainly cooked foods drains us of vitality and enzyme potential.

Some of the negative effects of food that's been cooked over 116 degrees Fahrenheit include:

- Loss of nutritional value caused by the destruction of enzymes and vitamins

- Loss of important microorganisms and bacteria that can populate the gut with good flora.

- Increase in trans fats and other obesity and cancer causing substances due to over cooking foods.

- Inflammation that can cause autoimmune diseases, contribute to depression and kick start rapid ageing.

- And much more....

So what can you do to stop piling on the pounds, start healing your body, mood and mind and start saving your life? The answer is simple. Stop killing your food.

Edible Sunlight

We know that sunlight is essential to all growth and vitality and raw foods, which take their energy from that sunlight, can then pass it on to your body. As long as fruit and vegetables remain in their raw state, those life-giving enzymes and that vital life force are still there. The moment those foods are cooked, that energy is destroyed. What was once a healthy substance becomes a substance that sucks the vitality out of your body when you eat it. This is why it's important to eat raw as much as possible. Living foods can nourish and support a living body. Dead, highly cooked foods create a dead, exhausted, lifeless body. In fact, according to Dr. Edward Howell's research, a lack or depletion of enzymes is the cause of aging.

Naturally Distilled

Another topic to remember when we talk about raw eating is that of water. The best thing about eating raw is that unlike with other eating systems, you have no need for a water distiller. The raw fruits you eat have already distilled the Earth's water for you. Your body is typically about 60-70% water while raw fruits are actually made up of about 80% water. Strawberries, peaches, oranges, broccoli, avocado, tomatoes and cucumbers are bursting with water and provide your body with pure, distilled, quenching water.

Another benefit of fruit is its action on the lymphatic system. The lymphatic system is a powerful circulatory system that can affect every part of your body. When the system faces toxic stress, the originally see-through lymph fluid begins to back up, change color and even solidify. This is known as interstitial constipation between the cells and can set the stage for many cancers. Raw fruit works on the system, much like a broom, cleaning out backed up lymph fluid and getting things clear and moving again

So you see all of the mind-boggling benefits of raw food eating. You may only be able to commit to a few raw, fresh & vital meals a week at this point. You'll still be able to begin reaping rewards without having to go totally raw. Pace yourself and remember that you don't have to decide to completely skip cooking. You can always lower the temperatures as close to 166 degrees Fahrenheit as possible and cut cooking times to save as many of those precious enzymes as possible. When it comes to leafy greens in particular, the less heat applied, the higher your dose of good-for-you vitamins.

In an ideal situation, you should be aiming towards 75% raw consumption. At this percentage, you'll start to see pains and aches you thought were with you forever disappear and the extra weight you've been carrying around for years will rapidly melt away. Most importantly you'll feel a sense of vitality, clarity and emotional balance that you never knew was possible.

By now you're probably ready to make the switch from dead to living food but how do you know what's good and what to avoid?

Have no fear. I've compiled a list of examples that will show you what to ditch and what to keep. (I'll be giving you even more lists like this throughout the entire book!)

Know Your Enemy

AVOID:

Do yourself a favor. If it's green, let it stay that way. Preserve the enzyme rich goodness of dark, leafy green vegetables and banish these supposedly "healthy" dead, enzymes-less foods from your table:

1. **Avoid Boiled Vegetables**: Boiling your vegetables forces their nutrients to leak out into the hot water and be lost. Also, because boiling usually lasts for at least several minutes, the vegetable's cells are completely destroyed and the enzymes which would have

helped you to digest and benefit fully from the vegetable are deactivated.

Example: Spinach is super-rich in nutrients like iron, calcium, potassium but when boiled, it loses its amazing benefits and you end up starving your body of the vitality it needs. Consider this: 100 grams of raw spinach contain 28.1 mg of vitamin C but when cooked it only has 9 mg. What a loss!

Replace with: When fresh and uncooked, spinach, along with other dark, leafy greens, forms the base of the raw food pyramid. Eat as much of it as you want in delicious tossed spinach salads and spinach wraps. The enzymes will remain intact and aid in digestion while you'll receive a full dose of the 30 milligrams of calcium, 0.81 grams of iron, 24 milligrams of magnesium, 167 milligrams of potassium, 2813 IUs of vitamin A and 58 micrograms of folate found in a cup of the leafy green.

2. **Avoid Fried Vegetables at All Costs:** Many people believe that vegetables are healthy, no matter how you cook them but this simply isn't true. If you're frying your daily sources of nutrition, you're unknowingly destroying all of the enzymes, vitamins, minerals and antioxidants your body is so hungry for.

For example, wok-fried broccoli: Broccoli, the powerhouse of cruciferous vegetables is completely destroyed when placed in the blaze of a searing-hot wok. That supposedly healthy broccoli stir-fry is actually wilted and depleted of most of its vitamin C and disease fighting abilities.

Replace with: Raw broccoli, marinated in diced garlic and olive oil. A delicious pairing that give the broccoli a sweet, slightly tender texture but leaves it uncooked so you can let your body absorb the phytonutrients like glucosinolates, powerful anti-aging and anti-cancer substances that make raw broccoli a must-have for your looks and health. Raw broccoli combats H. Pylori, a nasty stomach bug that can contribute to weight gain and anxiety. A cup of raw broccoli also contains an astounding 81.2 mg of vitamin C, 92.5 mcg of vitamin K and 57.3 mcg of folate.

3. **Avoid Long-Baked Vegetables:** While baked food is often said to be good for the health, the truth is that temperatures in the oven can reach very high heat levels quickly, passing 116 degrees Fahrenheit, ridding vegetables of both the precious enzymes and the many important nutrients they contain.

Replace with: A delicious raw carrot juice flavored with ground raw ginger and a hit of lemon for sharpness. 1 cup of raw carrots contain 21383 IU of vitamin A, 7.6 mg of vitamin C which can aid in burning stomach fat, 400 mg of Potassium to help combat high blood pressure, depression and anxiety and 2g of fiber to keep your bowel functions regular.

4. **Avoid Microwaved Vegetables**: Nothing destroys food like a microwave, especially when that food was once wonderfully healthy. Zucchinis are a super- food and require no cooking at all. Popular recipes like microwaved zucchini chips are an example of nutritious, living food gone horribly wrong. Once Zucchini is blitzed in a microwave,

more than 50% of its vitamin C, potassium and magnesium disappear.

Replace With: A gorgeous raw zucchini noodle or pasta dish. A cup of uncooked zucchini provides a whopping 21.1 mg of vitamin C to fight off aging, obesity and depression while its 0.2 mg of riboflavin provides vital cellular energy.

***If you're ready to really feed your body, checkout the deliciously fresh recipes at the back of the book! ***

The Takeaway Lesson:

If you take away nothing else from this book, remember this: **Dead foods can't sustain a living body**.

When it comes to achieving weight loss and a happy, healthy, stable life, dead, overcooked, under nourishing foods will only drag you down and hold you back. The first and most important change you can make is to dropkick these unhealthy foods and embrace living, enzyme rich meals to start looking, feeling and living better right now.

In Chapter 2, we'll deal with a substance so toxic to your weight, health and mood that it's practically poisonous. Plus, one simple change you can make to lose up to 6 pounds by the end of the week!

Chapter 2

Crystals of Death

Your body's deadliest enemy is not some lethal disease with a long, unpronounceable name. It's a perfectly safe-looking item that is probably sitting in your kitchen cabinets right now. If you have a mug on your desk, it's probably in there too. If you're eating or drinking it as you read these words, I've got some scary news for you:

Your body is slowly dying.

So what is this deadly poison that is legally killing billions of people worldwide? It's Sugar. That's right. Those innocent looking white crystals are literally the stuff that death is made of. "You're exaggerating!" You may say "I've been eating and drinking sugar all my life and I'm still here." And that, my friend, is the scariest thing about sugar. It kills us so slowly that we barely notice and so sweetly that we don't want to notice.

Killing You Sweetly

Sugar is mankind's biggest health enemy. It's been linked to over 141different diseases, disorders and dysfunctions of the human body. Despite this, the average American ingests more than 150 pounds of sugar every year!

From making eyes more susceptible to degeneration to promoting diabetes-related gangrene rotting in the feet, white refined sugar is a head to toe killer. And remember those precious, life-giving enzymes we learned about in chapter 1? Well, refined sugar can block the activity of our bodies' digestive enzymes and totally ruin them. The result is that instead of being digested by these vital enzymes, sugar just sits inside of the body, festering and rotting, making us fat, unhappy and seriously sick

If that's not a toxin, I don't know what is! But wait, you may ask, if sugar is a natural substance that comes from a healthy source (the sugar cane plant), then how can it possibly be so bad for us? The answer is simple. Raw cane sugar is natural. The sugars found in fruits are natural. The white processed sugar that we ingest these days is NOT. Refined white sugar is the result of a toxic process that includes the use of many deadly chemicals.

After the refinement process, what was once healthy raw sugar is now a frightening white poison completely stripped of all the vitamins, minerals and nutrients that it used to have. Just take a look at a small sampling of the many ways sugar is slowly killing us:

<u>Weight</u>

- Sugar encourages obesity.

- Sugar can increase appetite and food intake, causing rapid weight gain.

- Sugar can cause insulin resistance, which tells our body to store fat instead of burning it. This makes it difficult to lose weight.

- Sugar causes intense cravings & food addictions, meaning that it becomes impossible to just "Say No".

Mood & Mind

- Sugar causes major highs and lows in glucose levels, causing feelings of depression, irritation & weepiness.

- Sugar contributes to anxiety by sucking up our bodies' supplies of mood stabilizer vitamin B.

- Sugar has been linked with worse outcomes for disorders like schizophrenia.

- Sugar can cause Alzheimer's disease.

- Sugar reduces the mind's ability to learn.

- When sugar is given intravenously, it can cut off oxygen supply to the brain!

Health

- Sugar can enlarge and permanently scar the liver.

- Sugar can attack the pancreas and is linked with pancreatic cancer in women.

- Sugar can be a factor in many types of cancers, from stomach to lung cancer.

- High sugar diets have been linked to cardiovascular disease.

- Sugar speeds up pre-mature aging.

- Sugar is actually linked to cell death.

- And so many more frightening effects.....

Sugar and the Central Nervous System

High levels of sugar in the blood can lead overtime to neuropathy, the destruction of the nerves within the central nervous system. Over half of all people with diabetes suffer from neuropathy which brings with it several severe complications. When neuropathy is present in the feet it can even lead to the need for amputation to be carried out.

Sugar and Inflammation

Inflammation is the culprit behind many diseases ranging from cancers to heart disease and depression to obesity. Sugar is linked to a rise in inflammation. Here's how it works: When your body is faced with a heavy dose of sugar, it sends your pancreas into full-on panic mode, forcing it to put out too much insulin. This massive, unregulated rush of insulin is a recipe for increased inflammation. The brain is negatively affected too. A rush of sugar and the resulting inflammation has been linked to depression and even serious psychiatric disorders!

Sugar and Autoimmune Diseases

Autoimmune diseases, where the body is, in essence, being made to turn on its self, are reaching epidemic levels and research tells us we haves sugar to thank. When blood sugar levels reach high levels, the digestive tract becomes inflamed, causing tiny holes to emerge in the stomach lining. This is called leaky gut syndrome and thanks to the holes sugar has caused, toxins and even undigested food particles are allowed to seep out into the bloodstream, causing your antibodies to fight against what they believe is an attack. These antibodies then go on to attack your own organs in a haphazard and confused manner because they've been triggered to fight.

Everything from the thyroid to the eyes and skin are under threat from such attacks.

Very few people realize that diabetes is actually an autoimmune disease that is the end result of high blood sugar causing the body's own immune system to turn on and attack the pancreas, destroying the beta cells and stopping insulin production. In the case of multiple sclerosis, an autoimmune disease that affects muscle movement and vision, sugar can cause seriously damaging inflammatory molecules to be sent out from the immune cells. The facts are impossible to ignore: Sugar attacks your body and mind and can even cause your body to turn against itself!

There really isn't a book long enough to be able to list and explain all of sugar's terrible effects on the human body, mind and mood, but this small sample should be able to show you just how serious the sugar problem really is. If you want to shed unwanted weight and stay happy and healthy, kick sugar out of your life. This one simple step will rescue you from years of bad health and prevent obesity and depression.

The Sugar Challenge

Remember in chapter 1 where I mentioned doing just one simple thing to lose up to 6 pounds by the end of the week? I wasn't kidding. If you're interested in losing weight *fast,* this step is for you! All you have to do is ditch the sugar for 7 days and you'll be amazed by the weight loss your body can achieve. Do this one thing and without making any other changes to your diet &

lifestyle, you will see the pounds literally melt away before your eyes.

The numbers on the scale will plunge and friends, family and colleagues may start to notice that there is something different about you. You'll hear questions and comments like "Did you do something new with your hair?" or "You look different these days, good different." They may suspect you've secretly had some work done but you'll know that all you've done is this one simple and totally free thing.

Are you ready to take the challenge? If you want to start shedding pounds and healing instantly, read on for instructions.

Know Your Enemy

So what's off the menu?

Avoid

5. **Avoid High-Fructose Corn Syrup:** This hyper-sweetened version of sugar is found in everything from cookies to canned food. It may partially come from the corn plant but there is **nothing** natural about it! It's so sweet that even a tiny drop is sweeter than normal sugar and Americans are eating up to 60 pounds of it, each year. Created by a mercury–filled chemical process, this sickening syrup has been linked to cancer, heart disease, liver failure and dementia, even when used is small amounts. It can even cause you to grow fat cells around your heart! High fructose corn syrup has also been shown

to cause obesity at much higher rates than normal sugar. There is no safe amount of high fructose corn syrup to ingest so if you find it lurking among the foods in your pantry, throw this dangerous syrup out of your life before it destroys your fitness, health and mind!

6. **Avoid Jams and Marmalades:** You might think you're doing your health a favor when you reach for one of those all-natural fruit jams on the market. The truth is, the all-natural label can hide enormous and deadly sugar content. Added sugar in these products can make your weight balloon! Think about this: 32% of Americans are now obese as sugar content in food products keeps rising.

What are the risks? Added sugars can drastically slow down your metabolism. They can also attack and inflame your kidneys, throw your pancreas into panic mode and has even been linked to high rates of depression. Don't let the added sugars in these food products make you fat, sad and sick! Always read the nutrition labels and don't just trust the "all natural" label to keep you safe.

7. **Avoid Store-Bought Ketchups, Barbecue Sauce and Pasta Sauce**: Maybe you're not a dessert fan. Maybe you don't even like eating sugary sweets in the first place. That means you're safe, right? WRONG! Sugar is popping up in some ridiculous places these days and a food no

longer has to be a dessert to be swimming in the white stuff. A shocking example is store-bought pasta sauce, which sneaks an insane 12 grams of sugar into your body. If you go for the convenience of store-bought savory sauces and gravies, you may be eating pure, deadly sugar without even knowing it. The effects of these foods are even worse in many cases because when you don't realize there's sugar in your food, you tend to eat a lot more of it, leading to stubborn weight gain, hormonal imbalances and even infertility. Keep eagle-eyes on labels or consider making fabulous, sugar-free sauces at home. It will save your health and change your life.

8. **Avoid Many Salad Dressings: This is the secret reason why so many diets fail!** Nothing's worse than choosing to eat a salad for weight loss and finding out that you're dressing has as much sugar in it as a donut! The added sugars can bring terrible effects to your door, from painful constipation to blood toxicity and even death. Did you know that the rate of high blood pressure among children is now 4 times higher than ever? As children's fragile kidneys are coming under attack from the rush of sugar and overgrowth of fat cells it creates, this formerly "adult" disease is becoming common.

What's more, performance on IQ tests is slowly going down at the same time as added sugar use is increasing. Many researchers are linking this epidemic to added sugars as well. Added sucrose can even hijack your brain's processes. It impairs memory and learning ability by severely damaging your synaptic responses, meaning that your brain cells can't effectively communicate with each other.

Don't let added sugars steal your health, intelligence and weight loss success. Whip up easy and delicious dressings at home that will safeguard your weight and your well-being.

9. **Avoid Some Types of Breads:** It's a strange fact that added sugar in the form of high fructose corn syrup is now popping up in popular staples like pastas and breads. How can you tell if your bread has high fructose corn syrup in it? Use your nose. Because of its unbelievably intense sugariness, high fructose corn syrup has a tendency towards rapid fermentation. Your fresh store-bought bread will start to smell "alcoholic" or "beer-like" in just a few days, if high fructose corn syrup is indeed present in it. But what about the effects on you? Well, not only does this syrupy sweet smell like alcohol, it also causes the same damage to your body as heavy drinking. In fact, it has been directly linked to liver cirrhosis, a deadly condition that is

usually experienced by long-time alcoholics. It may be shocking to hear that your bread may leave your organs needing rehab but you can prevent this by choosing carefully at the bakery.

10. **Avoid Many Canned Goods**: Many widely available canned foods are soaked in sugar. A cup of canned tomato puree hits your body with a crushing 12 grams of sugar while canned corn guarantees you at least 5 grams. When it comes to canned fruit, the numbers are even more frightening. Canned pineapple drowns you in 25 grams of sweetness and maraschino cherries pour 41 grams of sugar into one cup!

If you make canned fruits and vegetables a major part of your diet, reconsider. Continually elevated blood sugar levels lead to diabetes and even blindness. Diabetic retinopathy can take place when sugar destroys the cells at the back of the eyes. Choose fresh fruits and real vegetables to avoid sugar's dangers.

Always read the labels carefully to find out which items contain added sugar .You may be reeling from seeing some of your favorite foods and beverages up there but not to worry, I've also provided you with some delicious swap-outs!

<u>So what's on the menu?</u>

- Raw Honey (Manuka and forest)

- Plenty of Real, Raw, Fresh Fruits and their pure juices
- Agave Nectar
- Stevia
- Coconut Sugar
- Dried Date Sugar
- Plenty of pure water(8-10 glasses a day)-eliminating sugar can cause symptoms of dehydration in the first few days so stay hydrated and be one step ahead.

I've left you some simple and delicious recipes at the back of the book, to help you avoid those toxic white crystals and see amazing results by the end of the week!

The Takeaway Lesson:

Sugar is little more than a legalized poison. The minute you start to remove it from your diet is the minute you start to heal and improve.

If you've begun your sugar challenge, I'd like to congratulate you on the awesome results you'll be seeing in just 7 days or less! Rapid and easy weight loss, stabilized mood, mental clarity and improved sleep are all on their way to you right now!

Now, join me in chapter 3 to find out which other foods have secretly been destroying your metabolism, ruining your health and messing with your mood and mind. You'll learn what they are and exactly what you can do to stop them.

See you there!

Chapter 3

All Carbs Are Not Created Equal:

Avoiding Simple Carbohydrates and Starches

One of the most important ways to lose weight and save your health, sanity and happiness is to understand the secret, deadly powers of simple carbohydrates. Now, that's not to say that all carbs are bad for you. In fact, every cell in your body needs to utilize carbohydrates for energy and they are your brain's only energy source. But not all carbohydrates are the same.

What Are Simple Carbohydrates?

Simple carbohydrates are simply put, sugars. They are composed of only one or two sugar molecules and are very quickly digested. This sudden rush of simple carbohydrates being ingested hits your body with a rapid overdose of sugar, causing many of the same problems that refined white sugar brings on.

Simple carbohydrates turn into glucose within your body, leading to, among other things, ballooning weight, a distressed liver and drastically fluctuating blood sugar levels. Simple carbohydrates have even been linked to life-threatening disease such as heart disease, breast cancer and diabetes. Additionally, they can up the inflammation levels of the brain, setting off a chain reaction that can leave you angry, anxious or depressed.

Cycle of Addiction

So we know that simple carbohydrates wreak havoc on your body and mind. Could they be any worse? Well, yes. The rush you get from eating simple carbohydrates can leave you with intense addiction-like symptoms when your body is deprived of them. Some have even likened this cycle to cocaine addiction!

Once you're on the simple carb rollercoaster, it's very difficult and a little scary to get off. Simple carbohydrates act in the same way as refined sugars, sabotaging your body by triggering powerful cravings for more and more sugary foods and making weight loss and fitness goals super-humanly hard to achieve. The simple truth is that the more of these health-zapping foods you eat, the more you will need to eat, just to feel normal.

What Foods Contain Simple Carbohydrates?

Know Your Enemy

<u>AVOID</u>

11. **Avoid White flour:** White flour is one of the most commonly eaten foods and this may be why its negative effects are visible in large portions of the population. So just what is wrong with white flour? Your body sees it as identical to white sugar. White flour causes your blood sugar to spike and plunge suddenly, like a faulty elevator. This leaves you feeling weak, hungry and drained. White flour has also been shown to increase weight

rapidly. It forces a rush of insulin and excess glucose is immediately stored as hard-to-get rid of fat.

12. **Avoid Breakfast Cereals:** Not only do these simple carbs cause weight gain, they also lead to tooth decay. They form glycoproteins which stick to your teeth, forming plaque. Bacteria then feed on these glycoproteins and destroy your teeth. Serious tooth decay can then lead to blood toxicity.

13. **Avoid "Whole" Grain Breads:** The "whole" grain breads being sold in many supermarkets are actually made mostly of white flour and sugar. This deadly combination stops fat from being used as energy, meaning that you'll keep putting on the pounds, no matter how hard you exercise.

Simple carbohydrates are one of your body's key enemies in its battle against the bulge.

What about Good Carbohydrates?

So now that you're ready to kick those sugary simple carbs to the curb, what should you switch them out with? The answer is long-molecule complex carbohydrates that will change your body, mood and mind for the better.

Weight & Health

On the flip-side of the carbs question are complex carbohydrates. They are nourishing, fiber rich and therefore, more slowly digested. They keep your blood sugar levels spike-free and are a great fuel for life, providing stable, long-term energy that won't leave you feeling suddenly wiped out. Even better, a helping of these good complex carbohydrates can ramp up your weight loss by significantly reducing your appetite and banishing those jittery sugar-cravings. Often packed with essential vitamins and minerals, complex carbohydrates are the good-for-you Jekyll to simple carbohydrates' Hyde.

Mind

And get this: Ingesting just300 grams of complex carbohydrates a day has been shown to help improve and stabilize mood, suggesting that they are safe and natural alternative to the toxic anti-depressants on the market!

With all of these body and mind benefits that complex carbohydrates boast, it's vital to make sure that they make up the bulk (or even all) of your carb ingestion. Check out this list of fantastic complex carbs that you can substitute in the place of those simple carbohydrates:

<u>On The Menu:</u>

- Leafy green vegetables
- Starchy vegetables like sweet potatoes, pumpkins, zucchini and squash
- Beans
- Lentils
- Peas
- Rich whole grains and products made from them

All of these foods offer the body real nutrition and revitalization.

So if you're ready to say goodbye to rapid weight gain, fatigue, depression and cloudy thinking, reach for the real stuff.

check out the recipe index at the back of the book for delicious complex carb recipes that will have you glad you left those powdered donuts in the dust!

The Takeaway Lesson:

Remember that when it comes to ingesting simple carbohydrates, your body experiences and deals with them in exactly the same way it does with refined sugars: Panic, inflammation, obesity, disease and depression

If you've already begun to eliminate sugar from your table and your body, you're probably seeing the weight melt off, so go ahead and boost your weight loss and your health even more by leaving those simple carbohydrates where they should be, off your plate.

In the next chapter, we'll blow the lid off the dangerous, manufactured food ingredient that is in EVERYTHING from beef jerky to ice cream and may be the culprit lurking behind all of your weight, mood and health problems.

Believe me, you won't want to miss it!

Chapter4

The Frankenstein Fats Your Body Can't Handle

Have you ever wondered just why eating most packaged, processed foods leaves you feeling off-kilter, exhausted, or plain sick to your stomach? The answer's in the packaging. If you're eating something from a box or a bag, chances are that you're ingesting deadly trans fats.

Trans fats are an unnatural substance that your body doesn't recognize and doesn't know what to with! They are created by food processing and are the end result of adding hydrogen to vegetable oil to help it solidify and have a long-lasting shelf life. In practically everything, from pie to pre-cooked poultry, cookies to pop-corn, trans fats are the bane of modern existence and have been linked to numerous health problems and conditions.

Trans fats are most notorious for raising levels of bad LDL cholesterol and lowering levels of good HDL cholesterol, leading to an enormously increased risk of heart disease. This occurs because the chemically created trans fats are so foreign to your body that your body's fat–digesting enzyme, lipase, can't help to digest them. As a result, they lurk in the blood stream, clogging arteries and causing massive heart attacks. Frightening!

Here are just a few of the other conditions and health problems trans fats have been linked to:

- Liver disease: They interfere with liver enzymes & upset the liver's balance

- Cancers: They prevent your body's enzymes from fighting cancer.

- Diabetes: They mess with the insulin receptors in your body's cell membranes.

- Obesity: They're linked to sky-rocketing rates of obesity and can lead to abnormally fatty & large stomach areas.

- Immune disorders: They reduce immune function and up inflammation levels.

- Asthma: They've been linked to asthma and allergies.

- Depression: They've been linked to a nearly 50% increase in major depressive episodes, even in those with no history of depression.

There is no good or safe amount of trans fats. If you want to control your weight and protect your health and mood, steer clear of these Frankenstein fats. Your body will thank you for it immediately!

Know Your Enemy

Here's a list of most commonly trans-fats containing foods to give a miss

Avoid:

14. **Avoid Fast Foods Such as French Fries, Donuts & Deep Fried Chicken:** It's well known that fast foods cause weight gain but while they expand your waistline they can also shrink your brain. Studies show that trans fats in fast foods enter your brain and replace the good fat there with bad fat,

causing brain cell death, dementia and a brain that actually shrivels!

15. **Avoid Non-Butter Spreads**: While margarine was once prescribed for healthy hearts, it has actually been linked to heart disease due to its trans fats. All trans fat containing non-butter spreads pose a serious risk to your heart's and your brain's health.

16. **Avoid Cake Mix:** As if sugar wasn't enough, cake mixes are also full of scary trans fats which are linked to infertility. In women who regularly eat trans fats, ovulation stops, making it impossible to get pregnant. These bad fats can interfere with your body's hormone expression ability, leading to thyroid dysfunction, menopause in women,

andropause in men and irregular hormonal fluctuations.

17. **Avoid 1-Cup Noodles:** Many people think of ramen noodles as a "better fast food" but in fact, the trans fats found in them have been linked to increased depression. This may be due to the way trans fats attack and inflame the entire body, with particularly disastrous effects on the brain.

18. **Avoid Items Containing Processed Vegetable Oil or "Hydrogenated Vegetable Oil":** These vegetable oils were touted as the healthier alternatives to real butter in the past decades but now research has found that they are in fact, heart killers. Cardiac arrest rates have risen mercilessly as hydrogenated vegetable oils have reached

peak consumption. The process of hydrogenation produces trans-fatty acids which wreak havoc on your body's cholesterol levels. More specifically, these oils cause your healthy HDL levels to plunge while spiking your dangerous LDL cholesterol levels, jump starting the process that leads to major heart attacks.

19. **Frozen Beef Patties:** Perhaps you avoid fast foods and other trans fats foods by preparing your own healthy meals. Excellent move. However, if your cooking includes using ground beef available at supermarkets, there's something you should know. These patties contain trans fats, making them dangerous to your arteries. A particular

concern is the shape of these fats. Trans fats are formed into an inflexible Z, making them the ideal shape to stuff your arteries and cause cardiac disease.

On the Menu

- Raw organic butter
- Coconut oil
- Raw fats in avocadoes, olive oil etc.
- Oven-baked (instead of deep-fried) snacks and meals

If you've heard (and felt) enough to make you consider giving up these deadly faux-fats, check out the recipe index for savory & nourishing recipes that'll show you how easy it really is.

The Takeaway Lesson:

Don't be discouraged, it's perfectly possible to live a life without the processed, nutritionally dead foods that trans fats are found in. Once you see your rapidly shrinking belly and feel your mood lifting, you'll be glad you made the change.

Psst...Chapter 5 holds a shocking "diet" secret you've got to read to believe!

Chapter 5

The "Diet" Myth

You feel like it's a conspiracy. You've been working hard to lose those extra pounds by only choosing diet foods and hitting the gym daily but somehow, you just keep ballooning! And looks aside, you've even been *feeling* less than optimal since you started your diet.

Well, there is something very wrong but thankfully, it's not with you or your metabolism. It's with those very same products you've been reaching for to help you get in shape. The simple truth? "Diet" foods make you fat! But how's that possible, you may wonder, when they say "low-fat", "lite" and even "reduced fat" right there on the packages? The short answer is that packages lie. Advertisers and marketers have come up with many slick tricks to keep you buying the same unhealthy, sugary, chemical packed foods in different boxes. One of the ways they do this is by using the diet food label.

When something is labelled healthy, fat-free or diet, consumers automatically believe it's a better choice but the fact is, it's often not. Check out the nutritional information on the back of any diet product and you'll be shocked and horrified. You're trusty diet foods are actually loaded with sugar, stuffed with saturated fat and practically leaking toxic chemicals!

Whether you're aiming to lose just a couple stubborn pounds or you're fighting to regain your health, so-called diet foods are your worst enemy in the war against weight.

Here are some examples that will leave you promising never to pick up another packaged "diet" food again:

The No-Fat/Low-Fat Scam: Products will have all the fat removed from them and replaced with...PILES OF SUGAR! The added sugar will harm your health and be quickly turned into stored fat that's hard to get rid of. Now that's what I call out of the frying pan and into the fire!

The No-Sugar Label: No-sugar often means that manufacturers have added in tons of saturated fats (sometimes trans fats) to make up for the lack of a sweet flavor. These kinds of items can have double or even triple the amount of fat that an ordinary non-diet option would.

The Lite Lie:

When a product is labelled "lite", it can mean several different things:

1. It contains less than a third fewer calories **or** half the fat of the original product.

This means that a product can have fewer calories but more of those *may* be calories coming from sugar or harmful trans fats .

2. It contains no more than half the sodium of the original product.

This means that a product *may* have less sodium but it could still be packed with sugar or bad fats.

3. It has a lighter color or even consistency than the original product.

All that this means is that a product looks different than the original product. It *may* have 10 times the sugar or calories but if it has a lighter color or texture, it can still be labelled "light"!

So how can you avoid getting cheated into cheating on your diet? It's Easy. Don't believe the hype on the front of the product, believe the nutritional information on the back. Read the fine print carefully to see how many grams of sugar, fat and sodium each product contains and how it stacks up against other products in the same aisle. You don't have to take manufacturers' word for your health. YOU have the power to protect your body by deciding what's really "lite".

Know Your Enemy

Here are some common diet-sabotaging diet products to steer clear of:

AVOID:

20.**Store-Bought "Healthy" Granola and Trail Mixes:** You're taking steps to improve your fitness and that includes healthy snack options. But when you reach for a handful of commercially processed granola or store-bought trail mix, this goal becomes harder to achieve. That's because these supposedly healthy choices are actually jam-packed with all of the sugar, saturated fat and even high fructose corn syrup you were trying to avoid. Consider the fact that a small bowl of granola without milk can add 500 calories to your daily total! Aside from the potential weight gain, granola, often consumed in the morning, will spike your blood sugar to a dangerously high level and drop it equally low. If this process is repeated daily, it can start your body on the road to a fatty, scarred liver, inflamed cells and even type 2 diabetes.

21. **"Diet" Foods Such as Flavored Yogurt:** Your morning yogurt can set off a chain of inflammatory events in your body. That's because if you consume even one small 150 oz. serving of flavored yogurt, you could be ingesting up to 20 extra grams of sugar. The

effect raises your blood sugar and can even lead to mood swings and depression. High sugar levels also cause the brain to become angry and inflamed, leading to brain matter destruction.

22. **Low-Fat Mayonnaises or Sandwich Spreads:** Manufacturers create additional flavor in these low-fat spreads by ramping up the sugar content. Often, they can contain up to 3 times more sugar than regular spreads and because they're always eaten alongside a meal, your body receives a double whammy of caloric and sugar content.

23. **Sugar-Free Cakes and Cookies:** With low-sugar options, the exact opposite of what

happens with low-fat options occurs. Manufacturers attempt to improve the taste of low-sugar desserts by pouring in loads of added fat. These fats are often of the trans fat variety which clog the arteries, inflame and depress the mind and are responsible for the obesity epidemic we are witnessing.

Don't leave your health and fitness in someone else's hands. Choose real, fresh and beneficial foods that will nourish your body.

***Create and enjoy real diet foods that are delicious, fat-busting and fraud –free, like the deliciously slimming recipe at the back of the book. Taking control never tasted so good! ***

The Takeaway Lesson:

You can't always trust the advertising but you can always trust your eyes and your body. If you've followed the steps this far, you can definitely make it all the way.

If you feel like something is blocking your weight loss, go all Sherlock Holmes and examine the "diet" products you've been eating for signs of a scam. You're more than worth the effort.

In the next chapter, I'll show you the dangerous way you may be packing on the pounds, sapping your happiness and hurting your health-all in one gulp!

Chapter 6

High Calorie Beverages: A Fast Way to Undo All Your Good Work

You may be hitting the treadmill hard, and watching every single bite you eat, but the roadblock to your fitness and health may actually be in what you drink. Many people feel like drinks somehow "don't count" and give themselves a pass to sip what they please, ruining all their hard work in a matter of minutes.

This is the single fastest way to undo your weight loss and health success and millions of dieters have made the same mistake over and over. It's important to remember that many beverages are actually just liquid calories, totally devoid of any nutritional use to your body.

When it comes to losing weight, it's all about energy in versus energy out. Unfortunately, some of the drinks that many guzzle daily are actually higher in caloric content than an entire meal! You may be doing everything right but a single high-calorie beverage a day can keep you permanently stuck at a plateau.

Think I'm overstating the case? Just take a look at these examples that are guaranteed to make you rethink that drink.

Curb Your Coffee Appetite

If you, like millions of others, can't imagine starting your day without a coffee run, you need to read this:

Many popular coffee chains' menus are loaded with an insane amount of calories. In fact, a regular 16 oz. milk and coffee beverage can range all the way from almost 200 calories up to a whopping 600 calories for certain whipped, flavored options. Just to put this into perspective, 600 calories is equivalent to more than 4 cans of Coca Cola! That delicious morning coffee is costing you the same amount of calories as more than 6 waffles or 3 breakfast burritos! Even worse, most of those calories come from sugars so you'll be left with a sugar crash that can leave you reaching for more of the same later in the day.

Steer Clear of Those Sodas

When it comes to your weight loss and health story, super-sweet sodas are the villains to your hero. They can be hard to resist, are extremely habit forming and make sure you pack on the pounds without even noticing. Ranging from 140 calories for the average can of soda to a mind-boggling 700 calories for a super-sized 64 oz. drink, these sugary options can trip you up on your journey to weight loss and health.

These drinks are usually made with high fructose corn syrup in the place of regular sugar. What's the difference? Studies have shown that high fructose corn syrup may actually be far worse for you. High fructose corn syrup has been tied to a higher rate of metabolic syndrome, a complex set of serious conditions including high blood sugar and blood pressure, an abnormal amount of fat stored in the stomach and high cholesterol. In addition, metabolic syndrome often includes serious depression, feelings of anger, tension and hopelessness, not exactly what you had in mind when you opened that can of soda, right?

It's also been linked with an even higher rate of inflammation than normal sugar and as we discussed in previous chapters, this sets the stage for diabetes, heart disease, autoimmune disorders and rapid weight gain.

High fructose corn syrup is digested much faster than table sugar and acts on the liver, forcing it into a distressed state known as fatty liver. This syrupy substance doesn't trigger our brain's "full" signal, so you can eat or drink it all day long and never feel satisfied.

The D-Connection

The final, frightening kicker is that high fructose corn syrup has been linked to reduced levels of vitamin D in the blood. Vitamin D is not really a vitamin at all but an incredibly necessary hormone that millions are deficient in. Vitamin D has been linked to reduced fat, particularly in the abdominal area and when levels of it are increased, inflammation markers go down. Vitamin D is also an acknowledged mood stabilizer that has been linked to a drop in depression, SAD and other disorders. Now do you really want to drink something that could lower your body's levels of this wonderful substance?

Pack in the Nutrition, Don't Pile on the Pounds

"Well" you may say "I don't even drink soda or calorie-loaded coffee. In fact, I only drink healthy drinks". If the healthy drinks you're talking about are packaged fruit juices and even some popular smoothies, I have some bad news for you. While plenty of fruit juices and smoothies are actually health and weight –loss stars, some brands and types are actually sneaky sugar traps that can leave you feeling worse, not better.

What's wrong with a nutritious glass of a vitamin-packed fruit drink? Well, that glass may not be as nutritious as you think. Thanks to new packaging technology, commercially prepared fruit drinks can sit in bottling plants for up to an entire year, waiting to be brought to your local grocery store shelves. In that time, the nutrients and vitamins in the juices are slowly deteriorating.

Many so–called fruit beverages actually have very few nutrients in them at all. In fact, fruit drinks may actually just be blended chemicals, sugar and water, with only a tiny drop of real fruit juice in them. They can contain the same amount of weight gain-inducing sugar or high fructose corn syrup as many sodas, not to mention a host of chemicals that ruin your fitness, health and mood.

How can you avoid this trap? If you do drink commercially prepared fruit juices, make sure that they're labelled 100% fruit juice and not "fruit drink" or "fruit flavored". And always check the nutritional information on the packaging.

Know Your Enemy

<u>Avoid:</u>

24. **Sugary Coffee Drinks:** The verdict is still out on pure coffee, with some highlighting its natural origin and high antioxidant content and others focusing on the jitters it can sometimes cause. But whatever your opinion, one thing is certain: The sweet, additive-packed coffee drinks at many popular coffee chains can spell disaster for your well-being. This is because when coffee is loaded with sugar, it behaves differently within your body than it normally would. When you ingest large amounts of sugar with caffeine, caffeine's natural tendency to raise blood glucose levels and increase insulin resistance

is heightened. This can lead to the "hunger effect" where the amount of calories you've consumed can't prevent you from feeling even hungrier. Avoid this damaging rush by enjoying real coffee and avoiding the high-calorie, sugary concoctions on the market.

25. **Sodas & Sweetened Energy Drinks:**

Here's a shocking fact: The average energy drink contains more than 20 teaspoons of sugar while a small can of coke exceeds the daily recommended sugar allowance by 10 grams! According to research, sweet carbonated drinks can increase weight gain by as much as 41% and that's not where the ill-effects end. Drinking just one 12 oz. soft drink can increase your risk of having a heart attack by as much as 21%. Whether you're worried about your waistline or concerned about your longevity sodas and energy drinks can destroy both.

26. **Commercially Processed Fruit Drinks:** Natural, full fruit juices are an important way to provide your body with the nutrients and enzymes it requires but store-bought fruit drinks are exactly the opposite. These drinks are merely *flavored* with fruit and are mostly composed of high fructose corn syrup, chemical additives and colorants. Their high-calorie content and unnatural mix of toxins make them a real danger to your body. In fact, research shows that consumption of just one commercially proccssed fruit drink a day is strongly linked with an increased risk for type 2 diabetes and cardiac disease. Give your

body the pure fruits it deserves and leave these dangerous beverages on the store's shelves.

<u>So what's on the menu?</u>

- Pure water (Never tap water!)
- Whole raw fruits that provide distilled water
- Young coconut water
- Unsweetened lemonade
- Green and herbal sun teas
- Fresh juices & smoothies

If you'd like to try mouthwateringly fresh fruit water that tastes as good as it is, the recipe index is all yours!

Juice Alert!

You've just learned some steps to help reduce your risk of unknowingly downing an unhealthy, high-sugar drink but if you really want to be absolutely certain of what's in your juice, it's best to make it yourself.

That's why chapter 10 of this book is dedicated to juicing and making smoothies. These two types of drinks can provide your body and mind with health, weight loss and mood benefits by making fresh, real nutrition available to every cell in your body.

Make sure you don't miss chapter 10, where we find out just why juicing and smoothies are so good for you. All this and more is only 3 chapters away!

The Takeaway:

Avoid the empty calories of bottled drinks and reach for life-giving quenchers instead.

Join me in the next chapter to find out which truly terrifying food items to skip in order to avoid obesity, chronic disease and depression.

Chapter 7

Processed Poison: Artificial Pleasure, Real Pain

Does the bulk of your diet come from boxes, cans or bags? If so, you may be facing a serious health crisis.

Commercially processed foods became widely available during the 1950's. Before the 1950's, rates of major health issues and diseases such as heart disease, cancers, obesity, childhood diabetes and even depression, were significantly lower than they are today.

Many researchers believe that dangerous, chemical-laden processed foods are to blame for the modern spike in ill health and unhappiness.

What's the risk?

Processed foods often contain dangerous additives that wreak havoc on your body and mind. With everything from toxic pesticides and preservatives to artificial colors and sweeteners included in the danger list, it's safe to say that nearly everything that comes out of a bag, box or can is a disease-causing processed food.

Here are some examples of common additives found in most popular processed foods:

Preservatives: Preservatives like butylated hydroxyanisole are meant to lengthen the shelf-life of packaged foods but ingesting them definitely won't help you to lengthen your life! Associated risks of this and other preservatives include increased cancer risks, ADD type behavior and irritability. Emulsifying preservatives are linked to inflammation and obesity.

Flavor enhancers: Flavor Enhancers like MSG (mono sodium glutamate) represent a huge risk to anyone who eats out regularly or eats a highly processed diet. MSG can damage and even destroy cells while also attacking the brain. It's been linked to Alzheimer's disease and migraines, among other things.

Artificial colors: The most commonly used artificial colors in big brand name foods have been linked to immune system tumors, brain tumors, cancers and extreme attention-deficit in children.

Artificial sweeteners: popular sugar substitute aspartame can attack the brain, destroying cells and can cause major weight gain. Sucralose wipes out your gut's beneficial bacteria and all sweeteners have been linked to depression.

Know Your Enemy

AVOID

27. **Avoid Most Packaged Foods:** Synthetic chemicals found in packaging and processing materials have been found to be leaching into packaged foods. These chemicals include formaldehyde, which has been found to be linked to a damaged thyroid. When the thyroid is damaged, your body can slip into a condition called hypothyroidism which is a

harbinger of major and stubborn weight gain. Aside from this, artificial flavorings and colorants have been closely linked with the development of dangerous brain tumors.

28. **Avoid Supermarket Bought Snack Foods Such as Chips, Cookies & popcorn:** Again, these items are a far cry from the whole, natural foods your body needs. An example of the dangers of processed snacks can be found in popcorn. This natural food is unnaturally zapped and then coated with a high calorie chemical "butter" flavoring. This flavoring has now been found to contain high levels of Alzheimer's disease inducing aluminum and other inflammatory chemical components.

Steer clear of the snack aisle and quench your cravings with honest, pure foods.

29. **Avoid Chinese Food Takeout & Other Restaurant Meals Containing MSG:** As stated above, MSG, or mono sodium glutamate is a brain attacking flavor-enhancer that is widely found in everything from children's snacks to Chinese takeout. It causes painful headaches and has been shown to up inflammation markers, sparking allergies and full blown autoimmune conditions in your body.

30. **Avoid Unnaturally Colored Foods:** Colorants are a toxic and unnecessary additive to processed foods. While natural fruits and vegetables possess appealing

shades, much of the processed poison on grocery store shelves does not, making the use of colorants widespread. They have a variety of dangerous effects. Blue #1 for instance, is a popular food dye that has been shown to cause kidney tumors while Red # 3 is a known thyroid poison found in sausage casings!

31. **Avoid Gluten-Free Packaged Foods:** You don't need them.

If you're suffering from the ill effects of gluten, it may seem like the easiest way to guarantee your health is to reach for a box from the gluten-free grocery aisle. But that's simply not true. There is no packaged food that's going to protect your health and the best things you can eat for your body are whole, real fruits and vegetables that are naturally gluten-free. Loaded with sugars, bad fats and chemicals, gluten-free junk food is still junk food so allow true healing by eating nature's own gluten free solutions.

Home-Made Fermented Foods: Nature's Finest Processed Food

Instead of these dead commercially processed foods, try a healthy processed food. That's right, I said healthy processed food! Fermentation is one of the most ancient food processing methods and if it's done properly and naturally, it creates some of the most life-giving nutrition you can find. Benefits range from the creation of beneficial bacteria to improved digestion, heart protection and allergy reduction. Fermented vegetable kimchi has been proven to increase weight loss by utilizing its good bacteria to control the appetite while raw kefir has cancer fighting abilities and unflavored yogurt's bacterial mix can combat inflammation and even diabetes. These are foods processed the way nature intended. Replace the supermarket chemicals with as many of these health–boosters as possible.

So what's on the menu?

- Whole, real foods that you cooked yourself
- Fruits & vegetables
- Kimchi

- Kefir

- Yogurt

- Homemade sauerkraut

***For a fantastic fermented kimchi recipe, check out the recipe index at the back of the book! ***

The Takeaway:

Ditch those modern processed foods and return to the ancient, natural healing of fermented foods. Fermented foods are a super-food that can extend your life, shrink your stomach and increase your health.

Check out chapter 8 for tips to avoid a major but widely eaten carcinogen.

Chapter 8

Processed Meats: Too Bad to Eat

Take a look inside your brown paper lunch bag. What do you see? According to doctors and researchers, if you see a salami sandwich, turkey ham slices or a hotdog, you're staring at certain death. That's because all of these are processed meats, one of the most dangerous food types in the world.

What's the Risk?

Other processed meats include sandwich meat, sausages, bacon, packaged ham and meat in frozen TV dinners. These processed meats become dangerous because a known carcinogen called sodium nitrate is used to cure them and help them to obtain a red, appealing color. But sodium nitrate has been directly linked to a major increase in cancer!

Sodium nitrate and the nitrosamines it causes to be formed in the body have been strongly linked with both pancreatic cancer and colorectal cancer. They've also been linked to cardiovascular diseases. While the current medical advice is to eat smaller amounts of sodium nitrate containing products instead of totally eliminating them, why would you want to risk it? The full danger of sodium nitrate cured products hasn't been completely uncovered yet but there's more than enough evidence of their fatal nature to steer you far away from them.

In fact, nitrates are so dangerous that they've even been used to kill off rodents! If that's not too bad to eat, I don't know what is!

Know Your Enemy

I'm sure you don't need more any more convincing, so here are some nitrates-containing foods to ban from your life:

AVOID

32.   **Avoid Hotdogs:** Research has shown that eating just one hotdog a day can increase your colorectal cancer risk by a terrifying 21%. The more you ingest, the higher this risk can climb.

33. **Avoid Bacon:** Swiss researchers have found that ingesting bacon regularly has been ticd with a high risk of dying from several cancers as well as heart disease.

34. **Avoid Beef Jerky:** Often touted as a high protein, healthy food, beef jerky is now known for links to raised incidences of diseases like stomach cancer and coronary heart disease. The risks are mainly due to the processing that the beef undergoes, raising its level of dangerous chemicals and putting your body in harm's way.

35. **Avoid Lunchmeats:** Eating just one serving of lunchmeats like salami can increase colorectal cancer risk by a chilling 36%. This is in part due to the smoking process that produces Polycyclic Aromatic Hydrocarbons.

36. **Avoid Smoked Fish:** Smoking fish creates these same conditions and can up your stomach cancer risk considerably. In addition, there is some evidence that smoked and preserved fish can contribute to the growth of harmful systemic Candida infections within your body. Candida sets the stage for autoimmune disorders and increased weight.

37. **Avoid All Meats Found in Frozen Meals:** While TV dinners are famously unhealthy, it's not always the caloric content that is your body's biggest risk. Nitrates are commonly used to cure and process the meats found in frozen meals,. Nitrates' carcinogenic properties mean that it's simply not worth

putting your body at risk with these convenience meals.

Now that you've just ditched that poisonous protein source, you'll need healthy proteins to replace it. Why not choose:

- Silky and super-satisfying protein powerhouses: walnuts, almonds and cashew nuts

Nuts are a fantastic protein-provider. They're literally stuffed with the weight loss –aiding substance. In fact, 100 grams of almonds have 21 grams of protein, the same as 100 grams of ham. And nuts are just as convenient on the go as processed meats. With everything from mood-improver magnesium to calcium for weight loss in them, nuts are the perfect snack and will have you forgetting all about carcinogenic cold cuts.

A Word on Soaking Nuts

While nuts make an awesome protein source, they need to be soaked before eating. This is because nuts have phytic acid, a substance that blocks your body from being able to properly digest them. Once you soak nuts however, not only are they more absorbable for your stomach, they're also beginning the sprouting process and thus, have become even more nutritious. It's a great idea to prepare ahead for snacking by keeping your favorite nuts soaking in an airtight container in the fridge. Change the soaking water frequently and enjoy the nutrients and taste of filling nuts anytime you choose!

***There's a recipe in the index for a quick Avocado Apple and Walnut Salad that can easily take the place of cold cuts in your lunch bag. Check it out for love at first taste! ***

The Takeaway:

While processed meats make for a quick, easy and high protein snack, the cancer causing nitrates they contain make them a vitality-vampire food to avoid. Switching them out for a healthier protein option is a smart move that will encourage weight loss, better health and a happier you.

In the next chapter, learn how a certain cooking technique can lead to everything from weight gain to dementia.

Chapter 9

Frightening Facts about Deep-Frying

Remember those trans fats we talked about in chapter 4? Well, they're not the only reason to steer clear of deep-fried foods. If you love the sizzle of food in the fryer, you're probably ingesting toxic substances that emerge every time you fry your food. These substances are known for causing:

- Inflammation
- Pre-mature aging
- Weight gain
- Diabetes
- Kidney disease
- Dementia

So what are these scary substances? They're called Advanced Glycation End products (AGEs). AGEs are formed when food is fried, smoked or grilled. Once you eat these substances, they stick to your tissue and light the fire of inflammation, making you sick, sad and fat.

Research shows that those who follow a typical Western diet that's full of deep fried foods, display super high levels of oxidative stress. This makes them look older, feel worse, and have a hard time keeping those pounds off. But if you're a frying junkie, don't lose hope just yet. Research also shows that those who switch from high heat cooking to raw eating or even the gentler forms of stewing, poaching and steaming make enormous improvements in their physical health and mental clarity. When it comes to weight loss, it's an amazing fact that without increasing exercise or changing the amount of calories ingested, those who cut out AGEs producing foods are able to significantly reduce the numbers on the scale.

Know Your Enemy

AVOID

38. **Red Meat Cooked at High Temperatures:** The Chemicals Heterocyclic amines (HCAs) and polycyclic aromatic hydrocarbons (PAHs) are created when beef is cooked using high-temperature such as when frying or grilling. These chemicals are dangerous carcinogens that can cause tumor growth in the pancreatic and colon.

39. **Full-Fat Cheese Cooked at High Temperatures:** The same cancer-causing components that are found in tobacco are formed when a high-fat food such as cheese is cooked at a high temperature.

40. **Full/High-Fat Milk or Cream:** When scalded or used in stir-fried dishes, these proteins develop the same AGEs that can compromise your health.

41. **Meat Substitutes Fried at High Temperatures:** Acrylamide is produced when starchy foods are exposed to high temperatures or an open flame. Acrylamide is an odorless white crystalline substance that is used as an industrial chemical. It's even used in sewage treatment but this harsh chemical

can also enter your body through high-temperature cooking. Its effects include neurological damage and it's a suspected carcinogen.

Replace these aging, fattening and carcinogenic substances with healthy meals that will delight your body and keep you AGE free.

So what's on the menu?

- Raw or lightly cooked fruits and vegetables
- Boiled grains
- Raw protein options like sushi & steak tartare
- Alkalizing lemon to undo the damage caused by AGEs

The Takeaway:

The fact is, AGEs are nothing to joke about. With a track record as major inflammation instigators, the list of diseases and disorders they cause is truly horrifying.

Instead of starting an inflammation fire with fried foods, aim for enzyme rich edibles that can put out the flames. Raw foods provide the food enzymes your body needs to recover from serious inflammation and revitalize itself.

Raw foods that are particularly loaded with enzymes include:

- Grapes
- Bananas
- Kiwis
- Papayas

- Dates

Add these liberally into your daily diet in order to combat the effects of AGEs and other harmful cooking substances.

Coming up in chapter 10, we'll take a look at the possible answer to your unsolved fitness and mood problems.

Chapter 10

Gluten & Allergens: Could They Be Causing Your Troubles?

Food is much more than mere sustenance for your body. It's a powerful substance that has the amazing ability to cure or kill. When you're eating optimally, feeding yourself with true nourishment and giving yourself what you need, you can SEE and FEEL the difference. Your skin glows, your body feels light and even movement is effortless. You breathe deeper, sleep more soundly and feel emotionally calm and balanced.

But what about when the food you're feeding your body looks like an invader to it?

Food allergies are a massive epidemic, spreading throughout society and targeting everyone, from the infirm to the strong and fit. While the causes for this are manifold and still largely unknown, there are steps to put out this fire. If you find yourself feeling continually swollen, fatigued, achy, depressed or moody, this may be for you. If you struggle with unexplained weight gain despite your best efforts to eat well and exercise, this may be for you. And if you find it difficult to muster the energy to get out of bed every morning but your doctor says it's in your head, this may be for you.

Finding out about a food allergy problem has been the first step to healing for countless people and has restored many lives.

Gluten: Grains Gone Wrong

Gluten sensitivity or the far rarer conditions Celiac Disease are not simply a popular fad. The consequences of eating gluten when your body is violently opposed to it are constant inflammation, thyroid destruction, autoimmune disorders like diabetes, obesity or wasting, extreme depression, organ failure and sometimes even death.

How Can Gluten Affect Me?

More than 55 different diseases have been linked to gluten intolerance or Celiac Disease. If you are sensitive or intolerant of the protein gluten, when it enters your body your immune cells will see it as a dangerous invader and will then mount an attack against it. This attack sets of inflammatory processes that can lead to the deterioration of cells and even organs in your body.

Gluten sensitivity is still a somewhat mysterious subject. It's not understood why one person has little reaction to gluten while another suffers terribly after just one mouthful. However, on the bright side, there's a fairly easy and inexpensive way to find out if your problems stem from this difficult to digest substance that is found in most grains.

If you feel the following unexplained symptoms:

- Fatigue
- Headaches
- Indigestion and Stomach Problems like IBS
- Unexplained Weight Gain or Weight Loss

- Bowel Problems

- Bruising

- Swelling of the Limbs

- Night sweats

- Rashes

Know Your Enemy

<u>**AVOID:**</u>

42. **Gluten and all Gluten Containing Products**

These include:

- Wheat and wheat products:

- Grains such as spelt, whole wheat, buckwheat, kamut, barley and rye and all products containing these grains.

- gliadin

- graham flour

- Semolina

- Matzo

- Bulgur

Be sure to avoid all products derived from these sources as well. Abstain from ingesting the above list for at least one month or more. Keep a diary noting how you feel with every passing week. Often, just two days away from gluten can clear the symptoms and pain away for those who are intolerant. If you feel no improvement of your symptoms, you're unlikely to be suffering from gluten sensitivity or intolerance.

What If I See a Difference?

If you do feel a major improvement after going off gluten for an extended period, it's very important to listen to your body's message. Testing for gluten intolerance is largely imprecise so if your body tells you that it feels better without gluten, that's all the proof you may require to continue with a gluten-free lifestyle.

If you do so, you are likely to find that your weight gain, fatigue and pain as well as emotional disorders gradually go away!

Other Allergens to Avoid:

43. **Avoid Peanuts:** Although nuts are fantastic and healthy foods for most people, if you're suffering from unexplained pain, weight gain or anxiety and have reason to suspect a food allergy, try reducing or eliminating them for a short time. If you do have sensitivity to peanuts, continuing to eat them unknowingly can cause the allergy to become more severe so an elimination diet is important if you even suspect an allergy.

   If not, what was merely sensitivity can turn into a major allergy that can cause major issues for your body including: swelling, eczema, sneezing, asthma, abdominal pain, and cardiac arrest. Anaphylactic shock, a dangerous and sometimes fatal condition in which your blood pressure drops rapidly can also occur.

44. **Avoid Tree Nuts:** One of the most common allergens, this allergy can cause everything from minor redness and irritability to life threatening reactions. If you suspect that you're in anyway sensitive to these, eliminate the food right away and contact a health care specialist.

45. **Avoid Milk:** In dairy allergies, the condition may be silent as with gluten. This doesn't

mean it's not severe but that you've become accustomed to the bloating, discomfort and pain that can come with it. There are tests for dairy intolerance and if it's proved that you have a lack of the necessary enzymes to process lactose, don't continue to subject your body to the pain and inflammation that eating dairy can bring. At the very least, eliminate the products until you have had a chance to recover from the worst of the effects. People who are intolerant to lactose have found major improvements can occur when they switch to pure, raw and unpasteurized milk products. If you are certain of the source of your dairy, this could solve your problems because dairy in its rawest form still contains the enzymes necessary to break it down efficiently for your body.

46. **Avoid Edible Fungi:** This food allergy, though rare, is common in those who have systemic thrush or candida. It's thought that edible fungi like the common mushroom can exacerbate a thrush infection and cause it to grow even more severely out of control. If you find yourself flushed, tired or emotionally disturbed after eating mushroom dishes, an elimination diet can work wonders and help you clarify the source of your issues.

47. **Avoid Alcohol:** This allergy again, is more common in those who have systemic thrush infections but because candida has become a

major health concern for so many, it's worth considering. This allergy is most often not an allergic reaction to the alcohol itself but to the source of or ingredients within the beverage. Some common allergens include allergy sparking histamines in wine and barley, hops or rye in liquors and beers.

You can tell you have an alcohol allergy if you experience extreme shortness of breath, nasal congestion, and nausea or hives moments after ingesting a small amount of alcohol. Elimination is the key here too, and you'll also find that whether or not you're suffering from this allergy, your health will make good use of the elimination period to absorb and use the nutrients that alcohol often leaches from your blood.

48. **Avoid Omega 6 Food Products:** These products include certain meats and many "natural" oils such as corn oil, sunflower oil and soybean oil. Human beings need an optimal balance between omega 6 and omega 3 fatty acids but in recent years, this balance has been thrown off kilter, and the ratio of omega6 consumption to omega3 consumption has become a lopsided 10 to 1.

These allergies are more common than previously imagined and if you have sudden onsets of asthma, allergies, breathlessness or sluggishness, consider eliminating the above oils for a short time and assessing your reaction.

This allergy is a particularly important one to sort out as overconsumption of omega6 products leads to system wide inflammation, producing results like arthritis and can even result in diabetes!

These allergens are common enough to make investigating your own immune response to them a vital and valuable step. In doing so, you are preparing your body for long lasting benefits and ensuring that the changes you make will have maximum effect. Remember, a sick, inflamed, allergic body cannot heal itself **UNTIL** the allergen is removed!

In chapter 11, we'll discover which trace metals and toxins could cause your body years of unexplained health problems and what you can do to stop them.

Chapter 11

The Toxin Protocol

Your body is an amazing dichotomy. Both strong and fragile, it deserves and requires all the care you can give it. When environmental toxins and heavy metals enter your delicate system, it is imperative that you remove and detox them as soon as possible. If not, the result can be headaches, nausea, foggy thinking and the worsening of any other conditions you may already have. Here's a list of the most common toxins and metals affecting health these days:

- Mercury

- Lead

- Aluminum

- Arsenic

- Cadmium

But What are the Sources?

Most of these toxins can enter your system through the environment but there are some foods which must be avoided to reduce exposure and to detoxify your body from previous exposure.

Below is a list of edible items to avoid.

Know Your Enemy

AVOID:

49. **Avoid Large Ocean Fish:** The sad truth is that our planet's oceans have become deeply

polluted with many industrial grade toxins such as mercury. Ocean fish, once a fantastically healthy source of omega3 fatty acids, are now a major threat to your health because of the large amounts of mercury they ingest from birth.

Because mercury slowly builds up in an organism, the larger the fish, the more mercury it's capable of containing. Mercury can cause everything from birth defects to lowered IQ as well as cardiovascular disorders. Mercury is particularly problematic as it can remain deep within the fatty tissue of your body and may take years to detox from.

50. **Avoid Refined Breads and Common Table Salt:** There is some debate about

whether aluminum is added to bread or is soaked into it during the industrial baking process which employs unhealthy methods and all aluminum mixers and baking pans. If you've ever scraped a finger against an aluminum pot, you know how easily this metal can come off its source and leach into your food. The one thing that is not debatable is aluminum's dangerous effects. It can cause serious memory and learning problems, dementia as well as liver inflammation and disorders of the heart and lungs.

NOTE:While the following are not as commonly found as the items above, they are a great next step to fully eliminating all metals and toxins from your body. Once you've eliminated the above items, you can turn to reducing or eliminating these:

Avoid Soft Drinks from Machines that Contain Cadmium: Cadmium depletes your body's available zinc and ingesting it can severely inflame the stomach. It can lead to extreme nausea, pain and fatigue and if ingested at low levels for a sustained time, can damage major organs from the heart to the kidneys. Because sodas sit in dispensing machines for an extended period of time, there's an opportunity for the cadmium in certain machines to seep out and cover the outer surface of the can. When you drink from this can, you are exposed to small but dangerous amounts of cadmium. In larger amounts cadmium can bring about sudden death so it's important to make sure your levels are negligible and that you detox your body regularly.

Avoid Canned Foods: Lead is linked to Alzheimer's, learning disabilities and anger and in larger amounts, it attacks the central nervous system. It can lead to comas, seizures and death. As mentioned earlier with other metals, lead builds up slowly and sinks into your body's tissues so that removal is very difficult. It's very important not to ingest canned foods regularly for this reason.

Avoid Chlorpyrifos Containing Foods: Chlorpyrifos is a toxic pesticide that is currently used on both food and non-food crops. It's been found to be incredibly effective at eliminating most pests and thus improving crop supply but its effectiveness is equaled by its toxicity. It attacks your body's nervous system by blocking an enzyme (called <u>acytyl cholinesterase</u>) that your brain needs to help you in controlling impulses. It can be found in peaches, apples and sweet bell peppers so eliminate non-organic sources of these foods.

Avoid Tetrachloroethylene Containing Water & Food: Tetrachloroethylene is an industrial grade toxin used in everything from dry cleaning chemicals to water repellents and fabric finishers. It can cause confusion, headache, dizziness and even death. This toxin is found in high levels in urban areas due to the close proximity with factories and in such cases, can seep into ground water and enters food supplies. If you suspect its presence, it's important to source your food and water from more rural areas and choose organic foods in any case.

Avoid Arsenic Contaminated Rice: Arsenic, a highly volatile chemical used in everything from pyrotechnics to pesticides has seeped into the ground water of many rural areas. This means that water-logged rice fields now present the risk of small amounts of arsenic in rice. If rice is a main staple for you, protect your body and brain from arsenic's effects by sourcing rice imported from non-contaminated regions.

Detox Protocol for Heavy Metals & Toxins:

1. **Eliminate Food Allergens**: This step is why we looked at allergens in the previous chapter. If allergens are not eliminated, every time you eat them, they will force tiny holes into your stomach's inner lining, causing an inflamed state that allows metals and toxins to enter your blood stream during detox.

2. **Have all Environmental Sources Removed**: This includes having mercury amalgam fillings removed by your dentist, making sure your water is not lead or cadmium filled and

eliminating commercially baked breads. Next, you can eliminate food sources of toxins by eating mainly organic produce.

3. **Heavy Juicing:** Green juices made from spinaches, kales and beets give your body a method to purify the metals and toxins that are stuck inside you. These greens cleanse the blood, aid liver and kidney function and attach to metals and toxins, pulling them out of your body in elimination. This step can be achieved by looking at the next chapter on juicing.

4. **Employing Saunas and Hot Lemon Water:** Regular use of a sauna will help your body force out the

toxins and metals through your dermis. The juices you drink will make the metals and toxins exit your fatty tissues and heat from a sauna can complete the job. Give your body extra detox support by drinking one to two glasses of hot lemon water first thing in the morning. This aids elimination of toxins through the urine.

Once you've reached the stage where metals are being loosened from your body, you've set the scene for true healing.

The Next Step:

You've come a very long way since chapter 1, and I want you take a moment to honor the commitment you've put into learning about your body, healing your body and eliminating so many of the poisonous substances that have been harming you. You've done amazing things!

But you haven't come all this way just to turn back now, right?

You want to keep obesity, chronic illness and depression at bay. You want to maintain your vitality with real, living foods and nourishing enzymes. You want to live a full, energetic, successful life without worrying about illness, aging or obesity.

Well, it's a good thing you've stuck around this long then, because here's where the major payoff comes in. At this point, you've reduced or eliminated nutrient destroyers such as processing, high heat, sugars, additives and others. We're done talking about what you need to avoid and ready to talk about the single biggest gift you can give yourself. This next chapter is about YOUR next chapter in life and the enzyme-rich, nutritional key that can unlock all the benefits you've been waiting for.

Chapter 12

Pure Vibrancy for A Brand New You: Juicing and Smoothies

You are what you eat. I'm sure you've heard that saying a thousand times but did you ever really stop to think about it?

It's actually a powerful statement of truth. What you put into your body **becomes** your body. So if you're throwing a bunch of sickening chemicals into yourself, you **become** sick. If you're feeding yourself nutrition-less, dead foods, eventually, you stop living.

But what if you begin to feed yourself with vital, potent, living foods? That's right. You become the vital, potent, fully alive person you were always meant to be!

Nutrients are the key to sustaining life and fresh-from-the Earth, raw juices and smoothies are the only way to deliver those necessary nutrients to your body in a way that makes them incredibly bioavailable to **every cell you're made up of**.

The importance of fresh juices in your fight to get and stay fit, happy and healthy can never be overstated. These fresh juices are your key to unlocking the millions of benefits hidden inside each fruit and vegetable. Did you know that there are still nutritionally beneficial substances inside plants that scientists haven't even begun to understand yet?

Think about that.

When you use these fresh, living juices properly, you are getting health benefits that science doesn't even know about yet!

When you begin to commit to a life of juicing, you don't just lose a few pounds here and gain a little more energy there. Juicing affects you on a deep-cellular level.

You literally change from the inside out until you are actually glowing with good health, life and joy.

No wonder those who start juicing never stop! Are you ready to give yourself this amazing gift?

Let's get started then!

Properly prepared juices are rich in inflammation fighting nutrients and vitamins, and often filling enough to do double duty as a quick and fat-fighting meal option, meaning that your excess weight will melt away with every sip.

There are two main methods for getting a burst of weight-decreasing, health-boosting freshness:

Juicing: Go Green & Get Lean

Benefits

Although juicing is currently a hugely popular trend, it's always been a secret weapon to fight the flab and restore balance and mood. According to the father of juicing, Jay Kordich, juicing allows you to obtain highly concentrated and easily digestible vital nutrient and vitamins that your body can use right away. When properly prepared, juices can produce an intensely nourishing and metabolism-boosting effect on your body. The fruits and vegetables have been separated from their thick fiber and pulp to aid absorption and Kordich advocates juicing up to a quart of vegetable juice daily. Dr. Max Gerson's healing protocol prescribes up to 13 daily glasses of enzyme rich fresh juice to help patients with serious illnesses. Dark, leafy green vegetables provide your body with various nutrients and aid it to rejuvenate itself. Leafy greens also help you to absorb calcium, a tested weight loss helper. According to Dr. Gerson's philosophy and research, juicing makes powerful enzymes extremely available, meaning that food is properly digested and utilized and your body is working at its optimal level.

Smoothies: Blend up Better Health

Benefits

Smoothies differ from juices in that they include most of the fruit or vegetable's fiber and pulp. They're a great option if you've already got good digestion and can handle the extra material. Smoothies include excellent fat-burners like quality protein, calcium and metabolism-revving vitamins like C and zinc which can help you control your appetite.

Different smoothie blends offer different benefits but in general their use of fruit with its fibers means that blood sugar doesn't spike suddenly, inflammation is prevented and you'll find yourself feeling full for hours afterwards. Smoothies containing avocado are a really great bet if you're looking to up your levels vitamin D as this silky ingredient is full of the fat-blasting substance. If you add raw cultured yogurt to your smoothies, your body is in luck! You'll get a dose of CLA, a healthy fat found in dairy that has been shown to really turn up your metabolism. An additional benefit of using smoothies for weight loss is that, as an easy, quick meal option, they cut out your desire for unhealthy junk food.

Guidelines for Juicing and Smoothies

- **Best Practices**: Because juices allow for a deeper and quicker penetration into your cells, there's a need to ensure that you're using the safest, most natural vegetables and fruits. While organic is ideal, it may not always be possible. In that case, go for lower pesticide risk fruits like avocados as opposed to high-risk kale and save higher-pesticide risk ingredients for when you can access organic varieties.

- **Add Lemon**: If you find the taste of darker leafy greens a bit overwhelming, remedy this with a dose of lemon. It takes the edge off and adds an extra shot of vitamin C.

- **Choose Well**: Fresh ingredients are the key to gaining the benefits of juicing. Make sure your fruits and vegetables look, feel and smell fresh and steer clear of wilting leaves and drooping plants.

- **Time is of the Essence**: When it comes to the bioavailability of nutrients, the less time between juicing and drinking, the better. Don't give your vitamins the chance to deteriorate. Only juice when you're ready to drink.

- **When it comes to Smoothies, There's a Meal in Every Cup:** Smoothies, with their full-fiber and high-nutrient content, can be excellent tools for weight loss. However, it can be easy to pour excess calories into your blender without realizing it. There's nothing wrong with a 500 or even 600 calories smoothie, as long as it is a meal and not a beverage accompanying a meal

And most importantly, have fun! You're embarking on an awesome journey and you should be proud! Be kind to yourself as you learn the ropes of this new lifestyle but always keep pushing yourself to reach your optimum level of health, vitality, fitness and happiness.

If you've made it to this point, you're already looking and feeling better. Believe me, this is only the beginning. Soon, you'll be experiencing all the incredible benefits of your hard work.

As you take your first steps towards the life-changing habit of juicing, allow me to wish you luck and please enjoy the juice recipes that have been carefully created to help you on your way.

 I raise a glass of green to you beginning the rest of your truly vital life!

***All of those irresistible recipes I promised are waiting for you.**

END

Recipe Index

The Ultimate Purifier

Serves: 1

Nutritional Information: Blood-purifying beets boast major dose of anti-inflammatory, enzyme protector betaine as well as immune booster vitamin C and betalin for Phase 2 detoxification. Celery offers vitamin K which boosts weight loss and fights metabolic syndrome while ginger cleanses and calms.

½ a beet

1 stick of celery

1 green apple

1 knob of ginger

Put all ingredients through the juicer

The Delicious Detox

Serves: 2

Nutritional Information: Cruciferous broccoli and kale aid liver to detox trace chemicals. Apples offer protective anti-inflammatory vitamin C while spinach contributes vitamin K for weight control and pineapple brings in a load of beneficial enzymes.

1 head of broccoli

4 kale leaves

1 cup spinach

2 green apples

1 cup pineapple

Lean, Clean, Green

Serves: 2

Nutritional Information: Apples provide antioxidant vitamin C, cucumber is quenching and cilantro and parsley cleanse the blood.

2 green apples

1 cucumber

1 bunch cilantro

1 bunch parsley

½ of a lemon

Early Morning Antioxidant

Serves: 1-2

Nutritional Information: Parsley purifies the blood and is rich in vitamin C, B 12, K and A, providing benefits that range from anti-cancerous to anti-diabetic. Apples offer cancer prevention in the form of antioxidants like vitamin C and celery provides anti-inflammatory effects from its store of luteolin, a powerful antioxidant.

1 cup of parsley

2 ripe apples

4 celery ribs

 The juice of 1 lemon

Stress and Fat Buster Smoothie

Serves: 1

Nutritional Information: Metabolism boosting raspberries and tryptophan rich stress-busters chia seeds are the main stars in this smoothie. Fresh kale adds mood-soothing magnesium.

1 cup of kale

1 banana

Handful of fresh raspberries

1 tablespoon chia seeds

Creamy Green Smoothie

Serves: 1

Nutritional Information: The creamy avocado adds a dose of weight reducing vitamin D and the apples add fiber while the broccoli provides vitamin A and K to help absorption vitamin D.

1 large ripe avocado

1 small green apple

1 lemon

1 handful of broccoli

Water, as per your desired consistency

3 teaspoons of raw honey

Wash, dice and blend all ingredients together. Pour smoothie into a glass and enjoy.

Whether you choose to juice or sip on a smoothie, going green will help you to start drinking in the benefits!

****

Sugar-Free and Seriously Delicious Recipes

Instead of a sugar drenched, processed or packaged breakfast, go for:

Hearty Breakfast Bowl

Serves: 3

Nutritional Information: Chia seeds are high in calcium which suppresses fat storage and magnesium which stabilizes mood and emotions. Cashew nuts also pack a punch with high levels of magnesium as well as vitamin B6 which has been linked to weight loss and restored energy.

1 cup almond milk

½ cup chia seeds

4tspns roughly crushed cashew nuts

1 large raw apple, cubed

1 large ripe banana, sliced

Dash of raw ground cinnamon

Agave Nectar to taste

Mix the ingredients in large bowl, top with a drizzle of agave nectar and enjoy a revitalizing and whole breakfast.

****

Sugar-Free and Seriously Delicious Recipes

Think salad dressing is a healthy choice? Think again. Many commercially prepared salad dressings are chock-full of sugar. For an indulgent, whole and fresh dressing that truly feeds your body, check out this recipe:

Decadent Avocado Dressing

Serves: 3

Nutritional Information: Avocadoes are highly digestible as they contain a large dose of the enzyme lipase. They also provide vitamin B6 which restores the mood, vitamin C which is linked to reduced belly fat and vitamin E for protecting the body's cells.

2 large avocadoes

1 large ripe lemon

1 small orange quartered

½ cup of water at room temperature

½ cup extra-virgin olive oil

2 teaspoons finely diced red onion

2 teaspoons crushed garlic

½ teaspoon minced ginger

Reserve the quartered oranges. Whip up all the other ingredients in a blender or mash by hand for a rich, chunky guacamole side dish. Sprinkle quartered orange pieces over the top and enjoy.

****

Complex-Carb Delights

Whole Grain Spelt and Sweet Potato Pancakes

Serves: 3

Nutritional Information: Sweet potato contains high levels of vitamin A which boosts immunity and vitamin C which is linked to decreased belly fat while spelt serves up a dose of mood–boosting magnesium and weight reducing calcium.

Serves: 3

½ cup of pureed sweet potato

1/3 cup of whole grain spelt flour

3 whole eggs

1 tablespoon baking powder

2 tablespoons coconut oil

2 teaspoons cinnamon

Dash of salt to taste

Combine whole spelt flour, baking powder, eggs, cinnamon and salt in a large mixing bowl. Mix thoroughly and fold in the sweet potato puree.

Heat a griddle, add coconut oil and spoon the desired amount of mixture onto it.

Let the mixture set before covering with a lid and allowing it to cook thoroughly before flipping.

****

Complex-Carb Delights

Forget those fast-food white flour pizzas and go for:

Quinoa Bell Peppers

Serves: 3

Nutritional Information: Quinoa is an excellent source of vitamin E which protects cells, magnesium which stabilizes mood, folate which protects against heart disease and zinc which prevents fat storage.

3 Bell peppers

½ Cup cooked quinoa

½ Cup mushrooms

½ Cup plain yogurt

3 Tablespoons olive oil

2 Tablespoons black olives

1 Large diced onion

2 Teaspoons minced garlic

Mix quinoa, mushrooms, yogurt, olives, onion and garlic together. Remove the cores and seeds of the bell peppers, rub their exteriors with olive oil and fill them with the mixture.

Place on tray and very lightly bake, keeping temperatures as low as possible.

****

Trans Fats-Free Healthy Temptations

Swap out those monster fries for this fantastic yam dish:

Garlic & Rosemary Oven Yams

Serves: 5

Nutritional Information: Rosemary and garlic both pack a mighty anti-inflammatory punch while yams offer fiber and heart-healthy potassium.

4 large yams

4 large tablespoons of olive oil

1 teaspoon minced garlic

Rosemary sprigs as you desire

Dash of salt

Wash, peel and cut yams into medium-sized wedges. Rub them thoroughly with olive oil and salt before placing in the oven to bake for 30 minutes. When thoroughly baked, sprinkle with rosemary sprigs and garlic and allow flavors to infuse before serving.

****

Trans Fats-Free Healthy Temptations

Skip those trans fats-soaked potato chips and choose:

Raw Kale Chips and Creamy Sesame Dip

Serves: 4

Nutritional Information: Raw kale provides big flavors and even bigger nutritional payoffs. It's rich in fat-busting calcium, packs a major protein punch and offers up brain-boosting vitamin B6 to boot!

Chips

1 large bunch of kale

Tear kale into chip-sized strips

Place in dehydrator for 24 hours at 100 degrees

Dip

½ cup sesame seeds

2 tablespoons lemon juice

2 tablespoons olive oil

1 teaspoon minced garlic

Blend all ingredients together well until smooth and creamy. Use as a dip for kale chips.

****

Gorgeously Guilt-Free Diet Food

Truly Diet Sandwich Spread

Serves: 3

Nutritional Information: Totally sugar-free, this spread boasts 20 different vitamins and minerals from the avocado alone, including vitamin E and K as well as fat melting oleic acid.

Vitamin C from the citrus and metabolism boosting capsaicin from the cayenne create an amazing weight loss helping spread!

1 large ripe avocado

1 small lime/lemon

5 tablespoons home-made hummus

5 tablespoons unflavored, live yogurt

1 shallot finely chopped

Dash of salt

Dash of cayenne pepper

Combine all items with lemon/lime juice and blend until smooth. Use this thick, creamy spread anywhere you'd normally use mayonnaise and enjoy maximum flavor without all that sugar and sodium!

Gorgeously Guilt-Free Diet Food

Raw Zucchini Noodles in Citrus Bell Pepper Avocado Sauce

Serves:

Nutritional Information: zucchinis provide your body a dose of antioxidant vitamin C, manganese for enzyme creation and bell-peppers give you an anxiety reducing blend of both vitamin B6 and magnesium.

Noodles

2 zucchinis peeled into noodles

Sauce

1 large soft avocado

1 small red bell pepper

Juice of ½ a lemon

1 teaspoon minced garlic

1 teaspoon minced ginger

2 teaspoons chopped red onion

Place all sauce ingredients in a blender and mx well. Pour sauce over raw zucchini noodles and enjoy!

****

Low-Calorie, Vitamin Packed Sips

You'll glad you gave sugary fruit drinks the boot for:

Apple Watermelon Fresh Water

Serves: 4

Nutritional Information: Apples are full of fiber and cancer-banishing vitamin A while watermelons are a great source of depression-fighting vitamin C and magnesium.

3 cups of sweet diced watermelon

3 cups of chilled water

1 cup of thinly sliced ripe apple

1 ½ tablespoons of lemon juice

Combine all ingredients in a blender and blend well. Remove the pulp with a strainer for a cool, clear drink or add the pulp for a fiber-rich experience.

****

Forget artificially processed foods and make a beeline for fermented wonders like:

Fantastic Fermented Foods

Simple Kimchi Recipe

Makes: 2 quarts

Nutritional Information: This kimchi is rich in vitamin C which triggers weight loss and protects the immune system as well as dietary fiber, to aid with digestion and elimination.

Large Chinese cabbage

1/3 cup hot ground red pepper

1/3 cup salt

8 cups of cold water

5 chopped scallions

1 cup sliced daikon radish

1 ½ teaspoons of minced garlic

1 teaspoon of minced ginger

1 teaspoon sugar to aid fermentation

4 tablespoons of fermented fish sauce

Combine salt and water and pour over the cabbage in large bowl. Press the cabbage down for 12 hours, using a weighted object. Remove the cabbage from the salt water and put the salt water aside. Combine the cabbage with all other ingredients. Put the kimchi in a large jar and cover with the rest of the salt water. Allow the kimchi to ferment for 5 days in temperatures no higher than 67 degrees Fahrenheit until the process is complete.

Fantastic Fermented Foods

Even More Simple Cucumber Kimchi

Serves: 3-4

Nutritional Information: This kimchi packs a potassium punch with potassium being linked to everything from lowering blood pressure to increasing fertility.

3 cucumbers

1easpoon of minced garlic

3 scallions chopped

1tablespoon cayenne powder

Dash of salt

1 teaspoon fish sauce

3 teaspoons sugar for fermentation

1½ tablespoons vinegar

Slice the cucumbers first. Then mix them with salt and leave to stand for 35-40 minutes.

Then, combine all other ingredients in separate bowl. Remove water from cucumbers and mix them with remaining ingredients. Cover and place in fridge for up to a day.

****

Love at First Taste-Guaranteed!

Who needs nitrates when nuts are just so much better?

Avocado Apple and Walnut Salad

Serves: 2

Nutritional information: Avocado offers vitamin E and D while walnuts lift your mood with magnesium and lime gives you immune system benefits with vitamin C.

1 large ripe avocado sliced lengthwise into strips

1 medium chopped up red apple

1 teaspoon finely minced red onion

2 tablespoons of pre-soaked walnuts

1 lime

Mix together all of the ingredients, top with a squeeze of lime juice and dig-in.

****

Feel free to mix, match, experiment and always enjoy your food. Happy eating!

END